# Cannabis and Women

*A comprehensive manual on how to improve your health, appearance, sleep, and overall well-being with the help of marijuana.*

Oliver Wrench

# Table of Contents

# DISCLAIMER

This information is not intended to provide medical advice or substitute for the advice or treatment of a personal physician. It is suggested that you get counsel from your doctors or skilled health professionals regarding any particular health concerns you may have. Readers and followers of this educational resource are responsible for any potential health consequences.

# Introduction

"Cannabis and Women" by Oliver Wrench reveals the complex and transformative link between women and cannabis through a ground-breaking investigation of history, health, and empowerment.

This captivating narrative goes beyond a simple historical account to provide a comprehensive overview of how cannabis has influenced and is still influencing women's lives throughout time and across cultural boundaries.

Wrench meticulously documents the various roles women have had in the cannabis industry, from the days of cannabis activism and legalization in the present day to the ancient civilizations where the plant was valued for its medical qualities.

The emphasis on health and wellness in "Cannabis and Women" is among its most alluring features. Wrench offers a thorough analysis of the ways in which cannabis has been utilized to treat health conditions unique to women, including mental health difficulties, hormone abnormalities, and menstrual discomfort. He dispels the myths and stigma that have long surrounded the use of cannabis by using personal experiences and empirical data to demonstrate the plant's potential as a holistic health tool.

Set off on an insightful adventure to learn about the strong connection between women and cannabis. More than just a book, "Cannabis and Women" is a celebration of the tenacity, inventiveness, and unwavering spirit of women who have utilized cannabis to improve both their own lives and the lives of those around them. Take advantage of the chance to read this engrossing and life-changing book.

# Chapter One

## Introduction

The words "cannabis," "weed," "pot," and "marijuana" are all specific to a singular botanical family that is well-known for its calming and sedative attributes. Nevertheless, the impact varies depending on the method of use, and it is forbidden in several regions.

The name "cannabis" refers to a category that encompasses three plants with psychoactive properties: *Cannabis sativa, Cannabis indica,* and *Cannabis ruderalis*. One of the most frequently used drugs globally is manufactured by collecting and dehydrating the flowers of these plants. It is often known by other names, such as pot, weed, and marijuana.

The name used for cannabis is undergoing modifications

as its legality expands to other jurisdictions. The term "cannabis" is becoming more commonly used to denote marijuana nowadays. There are some individuals who hold the belief that the name is more fitting or suitable.

While names such as "weed" or "pot" are sometimes associated with illegal consumption, the name "cannabis" is considered more neutral by others.

Furthermore, the term "marijuana" is seeing a decline in popularity due to its association with racial origins. The primary motivations for individuals to utilize cannabis are its calming and sedative attributes. It is also administered in many states in the United States as a remedy for various ailments, including glaucoma, chronic pain, and disorders of eating.

It is important to keep in mind that while cannabis comes from a plant and is considered natural, it may still have powerful effects that might be advantageous or detrimental.

# The History of Cannabis

The historical trajectory of cannabis is extensive and intricate, extending over millennia and including diverse civilizations and applications. Below is a concise summary of the significant milestones in the history of cannabis:

**ANCIENT HISTORY**

*The early utilization in Asia dates back to about 12,000 BCE.*

- **Central Asia:** It is believed that cannabis was initially grown in Central Asia. Archaeological findings indicate that ancient civilizations utilized cannabis for its psychotropic effects, as well as for manufacturing ropes, textiles, and several other goods.

- **China:** Cannabis was first used during the Neolithic Age in China. Hemp seeds and oil were consumed as nourishment, while the plant fibers were utilized in the production of clothes, rope, and paper. Cannabis was recorded in the pharmacopeia of the Chinese Emperor Shen Nung around 2737 BCE.

*The spread occurred across the Middle East and Europe between 2000 and 500 BCE.*

- **India:** Cannabis, also referred to as "bhang," was employed in India for religious and medicinal uses. It has become an essential element of Hindu ceremonies and is referenced in the Atharva Veda.

- **Middle East:** Around 1000 BCE, cannabis made its way to the Middle East, where it was used to get high by the Scythians, an Indo-European group of nomads. The Persian Empire used cannabis for its therapeutic qualities.

### *Introduction to Europe:*

- **Greece and Rome:** Cannabis was well-known in ancient Greece and Rome. Herodotus, the Greek historian, documented the utilization of cannabis by the Scythians. Its medical uses are also mentioned in Roman writings.

## MEDIEVAL PERIOD

### *Utilization in the Islamic World:*

- **Arab Health Workers:** In the middle Ages, Arab physicians like Avicenna wrote about the therapeutic benefits of cannabis. It was used to treat a number of illnesses, such as inflammation, discomfort, and epilepsy.

- **Africa Spread throughout Africa:** Cannabis was utilized for religious, medicinal, and recreational purposes in Africa.

# MODERN HISTORY

## *Colonial America:*

- **Hemp Cultivation:** European colonists brought cannabis to the Americas. Hemp was grown throughout the colonial era in America for its fiber, which was used to manufacture clothes, ropes, and sails. It was a significant crop in regions like Kentucky and Virginia.

## *19th Century:*

- **Medical Cannabis:** In the 19th century, cannabis extracts were first commercially available in Western medicine. It was used to cure a number of ailments, such as rheumatism, discomfort, and sleeplessness.

## *20th Century:*

- **Prohibition:** During the 20th century, marijuana was illegal in several countries. The Marijuana Tax

Act of 1937 essentially outlawed the sale and use of marijuana in the United States. The 1961 Single Convention on Narcotic Drugs, which designated cannabis as a restricted narcotic, carried on this trend internationally.

- **Counter-Culture Movement:** During the 1960s and 1970s, there was a revival in cannabis usage, especially in Europe and the United States, among counter-culture organizations. Around this time, the movement to decriminalize and legalize cannabis got underway.

*Late 20th and early 21st centuries:*

- **Medical Legalization:** During the late 20th and early 21st centuries, public perceptions about cannabis changed. The first state in the US to approve medicinal marijuana was California in 1996. Other states and nations followed suit, realizing the potential therapeutic advantages.

- **Legalization for Recreational Use:** Several U.S. states and nations, including Canada and Uruguay, legalized cannabis for recreational use in 2012, with Colorado and Washington leading the way.

## PRESENT SITUATION

### *Worldwide Trends:*

- **Legalization and Decriminalization:** Numerous nations and jurisdictions are now reviewing their cannabis legislation as part of a broader movement towards legalization and decriminalization. Growing awareness of its therapeutic advantages, its potential for commercial gain, and shifting public opinion are the driving forces behind this movement.

- **Medical Study:** Ongoing Research: Researchers are investigating the medicinal uses of cannabis, including its potential to treat a wide range of illnesses such as chronic pain, epilepsy, anxiety, and cancer.

The history of cannabis is complex and intricately entwined with human culture, civilization, and medicine. Evolutionary scientific understanding and cultural ideals are reflected in its trajectory from prehistoric use to present legality.

# Chapter Two

## Women and Cannabis: Historical Overview

Over the course of thousands of years, the relationship between women and cannabis has taken on several forms, ranging from cultural and social engagement to therapeutic usage and production. Here is a historical overview that emphasizes important points:

### THE PREHISTORIC AND MEDIEVAL ERAS

*Ancient utilization and cultivation:*

- **China:** Growing and preparing hemp for textiles was a common task for women in ancient China. The fibers from hemp were necessary to make clothes and other things.

- **India:** Cannabis (bhang) was utilized by Indian women for both therapeutic and religious purposes. It was included in Ayurvedic medicine, where it was used to improve childbirth and cure ailments including dysmenorrhea (menstrual cramps).

*Use as medicine:*

- **Egypt:** Cannabis was utilized medicinally in ancient Egypt. It was suggested to ease delivery and other gynecological disorders in a number of medical texts, including the Ebers Papyrus (c. 1500 BCE).

- **Middle East:** Women in medieval Islamic society utilized cannabis as a treatment for a range of illnesses, including gynecological disorders and monthly discomfort.

**EARLY MODERN PERIOD**

*Europe:*

- **Herbal Medicine:** Cannabis was mentioned in herbal medicine texts in Europe in the 16th and 17th century. Cannabis medicines were commonly utilized by women healers and midwives to treat menstruation issues and ease the agony of delivery.

## EARLY 20TH AND 19TH CENTURIES

*Medical cannabis:*

- **Western Medicine:** Cannabis extracts were first commercially accessible in Western medicine throughout the 1800s. Menstrual discomfort, migraines, anxiety, and other ailments were among the diseases that women utilized cannabis tinctures to cure. According to reports, famous people like Queen Victoria took cannabis as prescribed by her doctor, Sir John Russell Reynolds, to ease her menstrual pains.

## MID TO LATE 20TH CENTURY

### *Counter-culture and Criminalization:*

- **Prohibition Era:** Women and society as a whole were affected by the early 20th century criminalization of cannabis. But in the counterculture era of the 1960s and 1970s, women were actively involved in cannabis advocacy and usage as part of a larger movement for personal freedom and social reform.

- **Women's Liberation Movement:** Cannabis was used in the women's liberation movement as a social glue and a way to unwind, as well as a symbol of defiance against traditional customs.

## LATE 20TH CENTURY TO PRESENT

### *The Medical Cannabis Movement:*

- **Advocacy and Legalization:** The medicinal marijuana movement has seen a notable contribution from women. Advocates such as Mary Rathbun, often known as Brownie Mary, rose to prominence by giving edible cannabis to AIDS patients in San Francisco, thereby bringing attention to the therapeutic application of cannabis.

- **Health Benefits:** Anecdotal evidence and current studies continue to back the use of cannabis for a number of women's health conditions, including menstrual discomfort, endometriosis, and menopausal symptoms.

## *Leadership in Industry:*

- **Entrepreneurship:** Women have become more visible in the legal cannabis sector in recent years. Leading cannabis enterprises are led by women executives and entrepreneurs who prioritize creating products that are specific to the health and well-being of women.

- **Advocacy:** When it comes to cannabis advocacy, women are leading the charge to advance research, education, and policy improvements. The goals of groups like Ellementa and Women Grow are to increase awareness of the health benefits of cannabis and to empower women working in the cannabis sector

## CULTURAL REPRESENTATION

### *Pop Culture and the Media:*

- **Representation:** Sensitized images of women and cannabis have given way to more nuanced and favorable representations in the media and popular culture. More and more movies, novels, and TV series portray women as knowledgeable cannabis users and supporters.

### *Social media and establishing communities:*

- **Online Platforms:** Social media has given women

a forum to discuss their cannabis-related experiences, build networks, and promote legalization and awareness. Influencers and campaigners dispel stigma by talking about the advantages of cannabis on websites like Instagram, YouTube, and blogs.

Women and cannabis have a long and complex history that reflects larger social, cultural, and legal tendencies.

Women have been and will continue to play a key role in changing the narrative around cannabis usage and acceptability, from traditional medical applications to contemporary advocacy and industry leadership.

# Chapter Three

## The Cannabis Plant

The cannabis plant, officially known as Cannabis sativa, is a multipurpose and intricate species that has been utilized for its therapeutic, industrial, and psychoactive properties for thousands of years.

### TYPES

Generally speaking, cannabis is divided into three main types:

- ***Cannabis sativa:*** Known for its energizing properties and utilized for industrial hemp production because of its long fibers, this strain is often tall with thin leaves.

- *Cannabis indica:* Known for its sedative qualities, this strain is often bushier, shorter, and has wider leaves.

- *Cannabis ruderalis:* a less well-known and smaller strain with a lower THC level, it is frequently crossed to produce auto flowering strains.

## Key Components of the Cannabis Plant

The cannabis plant contains more than 100 distinct cannabinoids, the most noteworthy of which are:

- **Tetrahydrocannabinol (THC):** The main psychoactive agent that gives users a "high."

- **Cannabidiol (CBD):** is non-psychoactive and well-known for its anti-inflammatory, anti-anxiety, and seizure-suppressive qualities.

- **Terpenes and flavonoids:** They are compounds that give plants their taste and aroma, along with possible medicinal properties.

# Chemical Composition

A family of chemical substances known as cannabinoids affects the release of neurotransmitters in the brain by binding to cannabinoid receptors in cells. The cannabis plant is where they are mostly found. Tetrahydrocannabinol (THC) and cannabidiol (CBD) are the two most well-known types of cannabinoids. The following is a quick summary of the main cannabinoids'

**TETRAHYDROCANNABINOL (THC)**

*Chemical Formula:* $C_{21}H_{30}O_2$

*Structure:* THC is a phenol group-containing bicyclic molecule. The terpenoid backbone of this substance aids in its solubility in fats and oils.

*Psychoactivity:* The primary psychoactive component of cannabis, THC, is what gives users of cannabis the "high" they experience.

## CANNABIDIOL (CBD)

*Chemical Formula:* $C_{21}H_{30}O_2$

*Structure:* The molecular structure of CBD is comparable to that of THC, while the atom arrangements are different. It is a hydroxyl group with a bicyclic molecule.

*Psychoactivity:* Cannabidiol (CBD) possesses no psychoactive effects and is well-known for its possible medicinal benefits, including its ability to reduce inflammation and anxiety.

## CANNABINOL (CBN)

*Chemical Formula:* $C_{21}H_{26}O_2$

*Structure:* Degradation of THC yields CBN, a moderately psychoactive chemical. It has additional oxidation and a slightly different structure.

*Psychoactivity:* not as strong as THC.

## CANNABIGEROL (CBG)

*Chemical Formula:* $C_{21}H_{32}O_2$

*Structure:* THC, CBD, and other cannabinoids are all derived from CBG, a non-psychoactive cannabinoid.

*Psychoactivity:* Non-psychoactive.

## CANNABICHROMENE (CBC)

*Chemical Formula:* $C_{21}H_{30}O_2$

*Structure:* The molecular makeup of CBC is comparable to that of other cannabinoids, but it has a unique arrangement that adds to its own special set of effects.

*Psychoactivity:* Non-psychoactive.

## CHEMICAL CHARACTERISTICS AND EFFECTS

**LIPID SOLUBILITY:** Cannabinoids can readily pass

through blood-brain barriers and cell membranes because they are often lipid-soluble.

**INTERACTION WITH RECEPTORS:** As a component of the endocannabinoid system, cannabinoids mainly interact with CB1 and CB2 receptors. While CBD interacts with various receptor systems, it has a modest affinity for the CB1 receptors in the brain compared to THC's strong affinity for these receptors.

**SYNTHESIS AND METABOLISM:** The glandular trichomes of the cannabis plant are where cannabinoids are produced. They are converted by the liver into a variety of metabolites after intake or inhalation, some of which have pharmacological activity.

## THERAPEUTIC AND RECREATIONAL

## PURPOSES

**THC:** It is used medicinally and recreationally to relieve nausea, stiffness in the muscles, and pain. It also stimulates hunger.

**CBD:** It is widely utilized for treating chronic pain, anxiety, and epilepsy, among other conditions, for potential medicinal advantages without the psychoactive effects.

**CBN, CBG, and CBC:** They are being studied for their potential therapeutic benefits, which include anti-inflammatory, antibacterial, and neuroprotective properties.

Comprehending the molecular makeup and characteristics of cannabinoids is essential for the use of cannabis for medicinal and recreational purposes, as well as for the continuous investigation of its possible advantages and disadvantages.

# Terpenes

Terpenes are an extensive and varied family of chemical substances that are generated by a number of different plants, including cannabis. They may have medicinal benefits and are principally in charge of the flavor and fragrance of cannabis. The following are a few typical terpenes in cannabis:

**Myrcene**

*Chemical Formula:* $C_{10}H_{16}$

*Structure:* The monoterpene myrcene has a backbone of 10 carbons.

*Properties:* It smells earthy and musky and is well-known for its sedative properties.

**Limonene**

*Chemical Formula:* $C_{10}H_{16}$

*Structure:* The monocyclic monoterpene limonene has a backbone of 10 carbons.

*Properties:* It smells like citrus and is thought to have anti-anxiety and mood-enhancing properties.

**Pinene**

*Chemical Formula:* $C_{10}H_{16}$

*Structure:* Pinene is a bicyclic monoterpene.

*Properties:* It smells like pine and is well-known for its bronchodilator and anti-inflammatory properties.

**Linalool**

*Chemical Formula:* $C_{10}H_{18}O$

*Structure:* An acyclic monoterpene alcohol is linalool.

*Properties:* Known for its relaxing and anti-anxiety benefits, it has a flowery, lavender-like scent.

**Caryophyllene**

*Chemical Formula:* $C_{15}H_{24}$

*Structure:* Caryophyllene is classified as a bicyclic sesquiterpene.

*Properties:* It smells spicy and peppery and is well-known for its analgesic and anti-inflammatory qualities.

## Flavonoids

Cannabis is one of the many plants that contain a varied class of phytonutrients known as flavonoids. They have a number of possible health advantages and add to the plant's taste, fragrance, and color.

**Cannflavins**

- **Cannflavin A**

*Chemical Formula:* $C_{21}H_{20}O_6$

*Structure:* Cannflavin A is a prenylated flavonoid.

*Properties:* Its anti-inflammatory qualities are

well-known.

- **Cannflavin B**

*Chemical Formula:* $C_{21}H_{20}O_6$

*Structure:* The prenylation pattern is somewhat different but otherwise similar to Cannflavin A.

*Properties:* It shares anti-inflammatory properties with Cannflavin A.

**Quercetin**

*Chemical Formula:* $C_{15}H_{10}O_7$

*Structure:* Quercetin possesses a 3-hydroxyflavone backbone, making it a flavonol.

*Properties:* It possesses anti-inflammatory, anti-histamine, and antioxidant properties.

**Apigenin**

*Chemical Formula:* $C_{15}H_{10}O_5$

*Structure:* The fundamental flavonoid structure of

apigenin distinguishes it as a flavone.

*Properties:* It possesses anxiolytic, antioxidant, and anti-inflammatory qualities.

**Kaempferol**

*Chemical Formula:* $C_{15}H_{10}O_6$

*Structure:* Another flavonol is kaempferol.

*Properties:* It contains anti-inflammatory, anti-cancer, and antioxidant qualities.

## CHEMICAL CHARACTERISTICS AND EFFECTS

Terpenes and flavonoids have similar lipid solubility, which makes it easier for them to interact with cell membranes and increases their biological activity.

**INTERACTION WITH RECEPTORS:** Terpenes have the ability to modulate the effects of cannabinoids by interacting with both cannabinoid receptors and other brain receptors. Flavonoids frequently show their effects by inhibiting certain enzymes and having antioxidant properties.

**SYNTHESIS AND METABOLISM:** In plants, the phenylpropanoid pathway is used to synthesize flavonoids, whereas the mevalonate pathway is used to synthesize terpenes. These substances are processed by different body enzymes after consumption or administration, which adds to their pharmacological effects.

Understanding the structure and functions of terpenes and flavonoids is important for comprehending all of cannabis' medical uses as well as the entourage effect, which is when many of its parts work together to make the benefits stronger.

# Chapter Four

## Methods of Consumption:
## Advantages and Disadvantages

Marijuana, commonly known as cannabis, is a psychoactive substance produced from the cannabis plant. For thousands of years, it has been utilized for industrial, medical, and recreational uses.

There is a vast range of cannabis consumption techniques, each having advantages and disadvantages of its own.

Below is a summary of the most popular techniques:

### Smoking

*Methods:* joints, blunts, pipes, and bongs

- **Advantages**

*Rapid onset:* Results are usually felt in a matter of minutes.

*Control:* Dosage may be easily controlled by stopping when the intended result is reached.

*Availability:* This is the most popular and extensively accessible approach.

- **Disadvantages**

*Health risks:* may result in respiratory problems and expose users to toxic fumes from burning fuel.

*Odor:* It emits a strong, distinct odor that is difficult to mask.

*Short duration:* The effects usually last between 1 and 3 hours.

# Edibles

*Methods:* meals and drinks infused with cannabis

- **Advantages**

*There is no need to inhale:* there are no respiratory dangers.

*Effects that last:* Can provide relief for 4–8 hours.

*Inconspicuous:* This allows for consumption without drawing notice.

- **Disadvantages**

*Delayed onset:* It may take up to two hours to feel the effects, which might encourage excessive consumption.

*Dosage control:* risks of overconsumption due to difficulty in precisely dosing.

*Digestive problems:* Some people may experience stomach pain.

# Vaping

*Methods:* vape pens, vaporizers

- **Advantages**

*Healthier than smoking:* It limits exposure to harmful combustion byproducts.

*Inconspicuous:* It generates a minimal smell and is easier to hide.

*Rapid onset:* Effects are felt within minutes.

- **Disadvantages**

*Cost:* Vaping accessories can be exorbitant.

*Dependency on batteries:* Equipment has to be maintained and charged.

*Possible hazards:* There are worries about the safety of vape liquids and components.

# Tinctures

*Methods:* alcohol or oil-based cannabis extracts

- **Advantages**

*Rapid onset:* When taken sublingually, the effects start to show within 15 to 45 minutes (under the tongue).

*Convenient and discrete:* simple to use and carry without creating any notice.

*Accurate dosing:* simpler to regulate and quantify dosages.

- **Disadvantages**

*Flavor:* Some people may find the flavor unpleasant.

*Cost:* Compared to alternative methods, this approach might be more expensive.

# Topicals

*Methods:* creams, salves, lotions

- **Advantages**

*Localized relief:* useful for reducing pain or inflammation in certain regions.

*Absence of psychoactive effects:* not a high producer, therefore it's good for non-recreational usage.

*Simple to utilize:* straightforward skin application.

- **Disadvantages**

*Restricted effects:* does not relieve systemic symptoms; primarily helpful for localized ones.

*Differential absorption:* Depending on the product and the person, effectiveness may differ.

# Capsules and Pills

*Methods:* Ingestible cannabis capsules

- **Advantages**

*There are no respiratory hazards:* it prevents breathing in mist or smoke.

*Easy to use and concealed:* simple to transport and ingest.

*Accurate dosing:* precise and accurate dosage.

- **Disadvantages**

*Delay in onset:* Effects might take 30 minutes to 2 hours to manifest.

*Gastrointestinal problems:* possible pain in the stomach.

# Dabbing

*Methods:* Breathing in vapor from cannabis concentrates.

- **Advantages**

*High effects:* Delivers a powerful, short-lived high. Rapid onset: impact is perceived nearly instantly.

*Efficiency:* Minimal amounts are required to have a big impact.

- **Disadvantages**

*Health risks:* Dangerous chemicals can still be produced at high temperatures.

*Complexity:* This may be difficult for novices and requires specialized equipment.

*Strong effects:* For inexperienced users, this may be too much.

Users must select the cannabis ingestion technique that

best suits their needs, lifestyle, and health considerations because each approach has certain advantages and disadvantages.

# Chapter Five

## Benefits of cannabis on women's health and wellness

Cannabis has been examined for its possible health and wellness advantages, with several of these benefits being highly relevant to women.

**EASE OF PAIN**

- **Menstrual cramps:** Cannabis has been used to ease the pain associated with menstruation. Tetrahydrocannabinol, or THC, and cannabidiol, or CBD, are two substances present in cannabis that can help lessen menstrual discomfort and inflammation.

- **Chronic Pain:** Fibromyalgia, endometriosis, and migraines are among the illnesses that cause chronic pain for a large number of women. Cannabis, and especially CBD, has demonstrated potential in the treatment of chronic pain by interacting with the body's endocannabinoid system to lessen the feeling of pain.

## SLEEP AID

- **Insomnia:** Hormonal fluctuations, stress, or persistent discomfort can cause sleep difficulties in a lot of women. By lowering anxiety and pain, cannabis, especially strains strong in CBD and certain terpenes like myrcene, can improve the quality of sleep.

## SKIN HEALTH

- **Acne and Skin Conditions:** Due to its anti-bacterial and anti-inflammatory qualities, CBD may be used to treat acne as well as other inflammatory skin conditions. Products containing topical CBD can aid in lowering inflammation, swelling, and redness.

## MENTAL FITNESS

- **Anxiety and Depression:** Research on the anxiolytic (anxiety-reducing) and antidepressant effects of CBD suggests that it may be able to help women who are depressed or anxious.

- **Stress Reduction:** Using cannabis can aid with stress reduction. Certain products and strains have a reputation for being calming, which can aid in lowering stress and enhancing mental health in general.

## SEXUAL HEALTH

- **Libido and sexual enjoyment:** Studies have shown that cannabis can boost libido and improve sexual enjoyment. It may improve sexual encounters by lowering anxiety and boosting blood flow.

## HORMONAL BALANCE

- **Menopause Symptoms:** Hot flashes, mood swings, and sleep difficulties are among the symptoms of menopause that cannabis can help with. According to some research, cannabinoids may work with the endocannabinoid system to help balance out hormone abnormalities.

## BONE HEALTH

- **Osteoporosis:** Research indicates that cannabis may contribute to bone health and density maintenance, which is particularly critical for postmenopausal women who are more susceptible to the disease.

## ANTI-INFLAMMATORY AND ANTIOXIDANT PROPERTIES

- **General Health:** By lowering inflammation and countering oxidative stress, the anti-inflammatory and antioxidant qualities of both THC and CBD can promote general health.

## MANAGEMENT OF WEIGHT AND APPETITE

- **Regulation of Appetite:** Cannabis has the potential to influence appetite. THC is known to enhance appetite (the "munchies"), but CBD can help regulate it, which is beneficial for women who need to control their weight or who are experiencing an appetite loss.

Cannabis has a number of health benefits, but it's vital to be informed about any possible negative effects and the need for a proper dosage. Cannabis usage should be avoided by women who are nursing or pregnant, owing to possible dangers to the unborn child. Furthermore, local rules and regulations must be followed because the legal status of cannabis varies by location. It is advised to speak with a healthcare provider before beginning any cannabis regimen, particularly for people who are on other medications or have pre-existing medical issues.

# Cannabis roles in women's beauty and skin care.

Cannabis, particularly cannabidiol (CBD), has gained popularity as a component in cosmetics and skincare products as a result of its potential skin benefits. Here's how cannabis is being used for women's skincare and cosmetics:

**ACNE TREATMENT**

- **Sebum Production Regulation:** CBD can help regulate sebum (oil) production, which is a major cause of acne. CBD can lessen the chance of breakouts and blocked pores by stabilizing oil levels.

- **Antibacterial Effects:** As a dual-action strategy for cleaner skin, CBD's antibacterial qualities can aid in the fight against the germs that cause acne.

## ANTI-INFLAMMATORY PROPERTIES

- **Reducing Inflammation:** Due to its potent anti-inflammatory qualities, CBD can help lessen the redness and swelling that come with a number of skin disorders, including psoriasis, eczema, and acne.

- **Calming Sensitive Skin:** CBD can have a calming impact on ladies with reactive or sensitive skin, lowering inflammation and promoting an even complexion.

## SKIN BARRIER SUPPORT

- **Strengthening the Skin Barrier:** Skincare products derived from cannabis can aid in fortifying the skin's natural defenses against environmental stressors, including pollution and UV radiation.

- **Preventing Water Loss:** Trans epidermal water loss (TEWL) is avoided when the skin barrier is intact, which keeps the skin supple and moisturized.

## ANTI-AGING EFFECTS

- **Antioxidant Properties:** Free radicals, which cause aging, are fought off by antioxidants found in abundance in CBD. CBD can lessen the look of wrinkles and fine lines by scavenging these free radicals.

- **Hydration and Moisture Retention:** Skincare products with cannabis extract can help keep skin hydrated, increasing its suppleness and minimizing aging symptoms.

## HEALTH OF HAIR AND SCALP

- **Scalp Health:** By lowering inflammation, regulating oil production, and encouraging healthy hair growth, CBD-infused hair care products can enhance scalp health.

- **Hair Conditioning:** By deeply conditioning the hair, cannabis oil can enhance its manageability, luster, and texture.

## SKIN REPAIR AND HEALING

- **Wound Healing:** Because of its anti-inflammatory and antibacterial qualities, CBD helps hasten the healing of small cuts, scrapes, and blemishes.

- **Scar Reduction:** Over time, CBD may help lessen the visibility of scars by fostering healthy skin regeneration and lowering inflammation.

## TREATMENT FOR CERTAIN SKIN CONDITIONS

- **Eczema and Psoriasis:** By lowering itching and discomfort, CBD's anti-inflammatory and hydrating qualities might help treat chronic skin disorders like psoriasis and eczema.

- **Rosacea:** By lowering the inflammation and redness linked to this condition, CBD can help control rosacea.

# Chapter Six

## DIY cannabis beauty recipe

Making homemade cannabis beauty products can be an enjoyable and efficient method to utilize the advantageous properties of cannabis, specifically CBD, for enhancing the health of your skin and hair. Below are simple recipes for a variety of beauty treatments:

### CBD-infused bath bombs

*Ingredients:*

1 cup of baking soda

1/2 cup citric acid

1/2 cup Epsom salt

1/2 cup cornstarch 2 tbsp. of melted coconut oil

1 tsp. of water

15-20 drops of CBD oil

10-15 drops of essential oil (optional: lavender or chamomile)

Food coloring (if desired)

## Instructions:

- Combine the baking soda, citric acid, Epsom salt, and cornstarch in a large bowl.

- Combine the melted coconut oil, water, CBD oil, essential oil, and food coloring (if desired) in a separate small bowl.

- Gradually incorporate the moist components into the dry components, stirring constantly to prevent bubbles.

- When the mixture reaches a texture like damp sand, firmly pack it into the bath bomb molds.

- Allow the bath bombs to dry for a minimum of 24 hours prior to removing them from the molds.

- Immerse one of the bath bombs in your bath for a calming and skin-nourishing experience.

## CBD-Infused Face Serum

*Ingredients:*

1 oz (30 ml) carrier oil (jojoba oil, argan oil, or rosehip oil)

10–15 drops of CBD oil

5 drops of essential oil (optional: lavender or tea tree oil)

*Instructions:*

- Mix the carrier oil and CBD oil together in a tiny glass dropper container.

- Use essential oil, if desired, and vigorously shake to thoroughly blend.

- After cleansing, apply a small amount of the product to your face and gently massage it into your skin.

## CBD-infused body lotion.

*Ingredients:*

1/2 cup of shea butter

1/2 cup of coconut oil1/4 cup of CBD oil

10-15 drops of essential oil (optional: peppermint or eucalyptus)

*Instructions:*

- Heat the shea butter and coconut oil together in a double boiler over low heat until they are completely melted.

- Take the mixture off the heat and allow it to cool a bit before adding the CBD oil and essential oil.

- Transfer the mixture into a clean jar or container and allow it to solidify at ambient temperature.

- Use as necessary to moisturize and calm the skin.

## CBD Hand Massage Cream

*Ingredients:*

1/2 cup of shea butter

1/4 cup of coconut oil

1/4 cup of almond oil

20 drops of CBD oil

10 drops of essential oil (optional: lavender or rosemary)

*Instructions:*

- Heat the shea butter and coconut oil together in a double boiler on low heat until they become liquid.

- Take the mixture off the heat and add the almond

oil, CBD oil, and essential oil by stirring.

- Transfer the mixture into a container and let it cool and harden.

- Apply as necessary to moisturize and soothe dry hands.

## CBD-infused foot soak

*Ingredients:*

1 cup of Epsom salt

1/2 cup of sea salt

1/4 cup of baking soda

15-20 drops of CBD oil

10 drops of essential oil (optional: peppermint or eucalyptus)

*Instructions:*

- Mix all the dried ingredients in a container.

- Combine the CBD oil and essential oil, ensuring they are fully mixed.

- Place it in a container that is tightly sealed to prevent air from entering.

- Add 1/4 cup of the mixture to warm water and immerse your feet for a duration of 20–30 minutes.

## CBD-infused Hair Mask

*Ingredients:*

2 tbsp. coconut oil

1 tbsp. olive oil

10–15 drops of CBD oil

1 egg yolk (optional, for additional nutrients)

*Instructions:*

- Blend the coconut oil, olive oil, and CBD oil in a bowl.

- Add the egg yolk, if desired, and blend it completely.

- Apply the mask to dry hair, specifically targeting the ends and any areas that are damaged.

- Let it sit on your hair for 30 to 60 minutes, then rinse it off and cleanse it with shampoo and conditioner.

## CBD-Infused Lip Balm

*Ingredients:*

2 tbsp. of beeswax pellets

2 tbsp. of coconut oil

1 tbsp. of shea butter

10–15 drops of CBD oil

5 drops of essential oil (optional: peppermint or vanilla)

## *Instructions:*

- Heat the beeswax, coconut oil, and shea butter together in a double boiler on a low flame until they become liquid.

- Take the mixture off the heat and add the CBD oil and essential oil by stirring.

- Transfer the mixture into lip balm tubes or small containers.

- Allow it to cool and harden before using.

## CBD-Enriched Exfoliating Sugar Scrub

## *Ingredients:*

1 cup of granulated sugar

1/2 cup of coconut oil (melted)

15-20 drops of CBD oil

10 drops of essential oil (optional: lemon or orange)

## *Instructions:*

- Mix the sugar and coconut oil in a mixing dish.

- Combine the CBD oil and essential oil, stirring thoroughly.

- Place the scrub in an airtight container.

- Use it in a shower for the purpose of exfoliating and hydrating your skin.

## **CBD-infused Facial Cleanser**

### *Ingredients:*

1/2 cup of witch hazel

1/4 cup of distilled water

10–15 drops of CBD oil 5 drops of essential oil (optional: tea tree or lavender)

*Instructions:*

- Combine all the ingredients in a small bottle.

- Ensure thorough mixing by vigorously shaking before each use.

- Apply the product to your face using a cotton pad after you have cleansed your skin.

These homemade beauty products infused with CBD can be personalized with your preferred essential oils and ingredients to match your preferences and skin type. It is essential to conduct a patch test prior to applying a new product, particularly if you have sensitive skin.

# Beauty Products

**Superior Ingredient Quality:** Utilize premium-grade, unadulterated CBD oil and additional organic components to guarantee optimal outcomes.

**Patch Test:** It is crucial to conduct a patch test with new components to detect any negative responses, particularly if you have sensitive skin.

**Storage:** Preserve the efficacy and avoid degradation of your DIY items by storing them in dark, cool locations.

By creating your own beauty products infused with cannabis, you have the ability to tailor them to your specific preferences and experience the inherent advantages of cannabis for your skin and hair.

# Chapter Seven

## Cannabis and Pregnancy

Cannabis usage during pregnancy is a source of great concern owing to the risks it could pose to both the mother and the developing fetus.

The potential hazards of consuming cannabis during pregnancy are worth considering.

**DEVELOPMENTAL PROBLEMS:**

- *Cognitive and Behavioral Effects:* Research indicates that cannabis exposure during pregnancy may impact the developing fetus's brain, which may result in behavioral and cognitive problems in later life. This covers issues with focus, memory, and problem-solving abilities.

- *Low Birth Weight:* Pregnancy-related cannabis use

has been linked to lower birth weights, which may result in further health issues for the unborn child.

## PREMATURE BIRTH:

- *Premature Delivery:* Research suggests that cannabis usage may raise the risk of premature birth, which can have a variety of negative health effects on the unborn child.

## NEONATAL PERFORMANCE:

- *Increased NICU Admissions:* Due to a variety of health issues, infants who are exposed to cannabis while still in utero are more likely to be admitted to neonatal intensive care units (NICU).

## PLACENTAL PROBLEMS:

- *Placental Insufficiency:* The use of cannabis may have an impact on placental function, which is essential for supplying the growing fetus with nutrition and oxygen.

## RESPIRATORY ISSUES:

- *Secondhand Smoke:* If cannabis is smoked, the mother and the growing fetus may be at risk for respiratory problems if they inhale smoke, especially secondhand smoke.

## Guidelines and suggestions

## MEDICAL GUIDANCE:

- *Consult Healthcare practitioners:* Before consuming cannabis, women who are pregnant or intend to become pregnant should speak with their healthcare practitioners. This involves talking about any current medication use and thinking about different options for treating ailments like pain, anxiety, or nausea.

## AVOIDING USE:

- *No Safe Amount:* Using cannabis while pregnant is not known to be safe in any amount. As a result, it is usually advised to abstain from cannabis completely during this time.

## ALTERNATIVE MEDICAL MEASURES:

- *Non-Cannabis Treatments:* Medical professionals can suggest safer, non-cannabis treatments that are better researched and comprehended in the context of pregnancy for ailments like pain or morning sickness.

Pregnant women should refrain from using cannabis due to the potential hazards and the absence of conclusive data about its safe usage. Healthcare practitioners have a vital responsibility in teaching and assisting women to guarantee the health and well-being of both the mother and the developing baby. If you are currently pregnant or intending to conceive and are consuming cannabis, it is crucial to consult with a healthcare practitioner in order to find safer options and obtain suitable advice.

# ACKNOWLEDGEMENTS

God alone is worthy of all praise. In addition, I would like to express my gratitude to my amazing family, partner, readers, fans, friends, and customers for their unwavering encouragement and support.

www.ingramcontent.com/pod-product-compliance
Lightning Source LLC
Chambersburg PA
CBHW031134020426
42333CB00012B/366